LI

H

TiPS

LINDA BUTTLE

LITTLE BOOK OF
HAIR TIPS

LINDA BUTTLE

Ruby BOOKS

Ruby Books
Scarborough House
29 James Street West
Bath BA1 2BT

Phone 44 (0) 1225 316013 **Fax** 44 (0) 1225 445836
E-mail rubybooks@absolutepress.co.uk
Web www.absolutepress.co.uk

Written by Linda Buttle
The author has asserted her moral rights.

Designed by Blue Sunflower Creative
Series Editor Meg Avent

A catalogue record of this book is available
from the British Library

ISBN 0 9549871 1 X

Printed and bound by Legoprint, Italy

50 Fabulous tips on how

to achieve beautiful hair.

Always **use products** designed **specifically for your hair type** to ensure you get the best results.

2

Make it part of your regular routine to **partially dry your hair before applying** any **styling products.** The logic behind this is that products applied to wet hair will dilute their effectiveness.

3

Holidays are hard on your hair, so if **you're off to the beach** be sure to **pack a protective hair product** with a high SPF to ward of the harmful effects of the sea and sun.

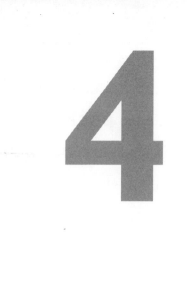

To boost flat hair, **blow-dry** with your head **turned upside down** and finish with a blast of cold air for **lasting lift.**

5

Using **styling products** after every wash will not only tame unruly locks but will also **protect hair from heat damage.**

6

After shampooing, **comb through conditioner** with a large-toothed comb so that the conditioner coats all your hair and removes any knots for **silky smooth results.**

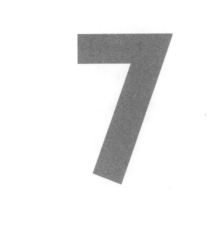

Revitalise dull locks with a detoxifying shampoo that will remove any built-up residue in the hair. Follow with a deep conditioning treatment and marvel at the difference it makes.

8

Having a **trim every six weeks** is the best way **to keep** flyaway hair and **split ends at bay.**

9

Hair looks glossiest when the cuticles lie flat. To achieve this, point the nozzle of your hairdryer down the hair shaft when drying and finish with a touch of serum.

10

Let your hair dry naturally as often as you can to keep it in great condition.

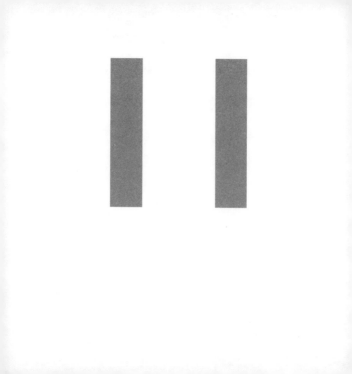

For **an effective treatment for dandruff** or an itchy scalp use a good quality **tea tree shampoo.**

12

Rinsing hair in mineral water may seem extravagant but for a special occasion it's a **great way to boost shine.**

13

To **combat static** hair, lightly rub a fabric softener sheet over the surface of your hair. It's a great quick-fix measure in times of need.

14

Avoid **crossing your legs** whilst having your hair cut, it will alter your posture and could leave you with an **uneven haircut!**

15

A **scalp massage** is not only incredibly relaxing but encourages good circulation and can **boost hair growth.**

16

Suss out a new salon by having a

free consultation

or just booking yourself in for a

blow-dry. If you like what they do it

will give you confidence

to go back for a full cut and colour

without the worry.

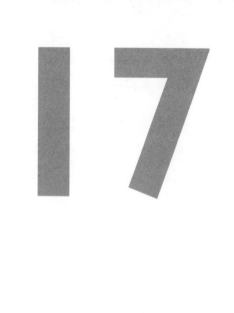

Don't overload your hair with products;

just add a little at a time until you get

the desired effect.

18

Avoid **piling long hair on top of your head** when shampooing as it **encourages tangles** to form, instead just let it hang down naturally as you wash it.

19

A really good cut

that's regularly maintained needs the

**minimum amount
of styling.**

20

Transform lifeless looking hair by interspersing lots of different colours throughout to **create an illusion of texture and movement.**

21

If you have a **sensitive scalp,** use delicate **non-perfumed products,** and get into the habit of rinsing thoroughly as shampoo left on the scalp can cause irritation.

22

It might sound scary, but **having layers** cut into fine hair **can make your hair look much thicker** by helping it stand away from your head rather than hanging flat.

23

Shine is created by light being reflected

off your hair, therefore the

smoother your hair the

better the shine, which is

why straightening irons are so popular.

24

If you **suffer from flyaway hair** made worse by the dry atmosphere caused by central heating, **switch to a leave-in conditioner** and see the difference.

25

Whenever you've **been in the sea** or a swimming pool **rinse your hair with fresh water** to avoid the drying effect of salt and chlorine.

26

Attaching a fake hairpiece is an

**instant way to update
your hairstyle,** ideal for a

really dressy look for a special night out

on the town.

27

A good old-fashioned, tried and trusted **trick for shiny hair** is to **rinse dark hair** with a mix of two cups of cold water and one cup of Guinness. **For blonde hair,** rinse in a mix of five cups of cold water and a quarter of a cup of white wine vinegar.

28

Add **maximum volume** to your hair by working a little mousse into the roots and then add height by **blow-drying with a diffuser** attachment.

29

Hair mascara applied to your parting or crown is a quick and easy way **to disguise grown-out roots,** a great pre-party trick.

30

If you need to style in a hurry, switch your hairdryer to a **faster speed, not a higher heat.** A faster flow dries your hair quicker and does less damage.

31

Adding **highlights** or lowlights **can break** up the **heaviness** of thick hair to give a softer more feminine look.

32

Poor rinsing is one of the prime causes of **dull hair.** A good way to get around this is to rinse your hair for twice as long as you think you need to.

33

Give your hair a boost with a **rich moisturising hair pack** whilst you're relaxing **in the bath.** The steam will encourage the moisturising ingredients to get to work.

34

If you're considering a **dramatic change in hair colour** always **ask the advice of a professional** hairdresser, especially if you have damaged or pre-coloured hair. They will also be able to suggest the best tones for your skin type.

35

Get rid of unsightly hair dye stains from around your hairline by dipping a cotton wool ball into milk and applying it to your skin.

36

For **super-sexy curls without unwanted frizz,** take two-inch sections and twist them before drying with a diffuser.

37

Regular exercise and a healthy diet are not only great for your overall health but will **keep** your **hair in tip-top condition** too.

38

To **combat oily hair** switch to a mild frequent-use shampoo and **wash in cool water,** taking great care to treat the scalp gently. Blot hair to remove excess water and dry with a low heat setting.

39

An **elegant chignon** is a quick way to put your hair up, perfect for **an instant evening look.** Simply backcomb for a little volume before pulling back into a ponytail, twisting and pinning into place.

40

The **quality of your hairbrush** is just **as important as** using the **right shampoo** and conditioner. Your stylist will be able to recommend one that is best suited to your hair type.

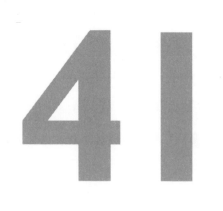

As hair is most **prone to heat damage** when it is nearly dry, opt for a **cool setting on your hairdryer** in the final stages of blow-drying.

42

Combing your hair prior to washing makes **tangles less of a problem** and removes loose hairs so they won't block up your plughole.

43

Salon training nights are a great way to keep the cost of your haircut to a minimum and **are sometimes free.** Just be sure to agree on exactly what it is you want before they start cutting.

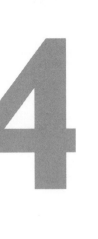

Your **hair is** at its **weakest when wet** so avoid brushing, instead use a wide-toothed comb.

45

To **straighten hair without costly straightening irons,** place sections of hair between two large round brushes and move down the hair shaft as you blow-dry it, keeping the hair taut at all times.

46

If you've **run out of conditioner use a body moisturiser** instead that will act like a leave-in conditioner. Likewise, a little sun cream works well in hot weather if you've left your hair protection spray at home.

When choosing from a wealth of styling products, it's good to remember that **gel works better on curly hair,** whilst mousse is best for adding body to fine hair.

48

Lemon juice and camomile tea are **natural highlighers** on blonde and fair hair. Simply mix the juice of a lemon with two cups of camomile tea (brewed and cooled), pour over your hair and sit in the sun. Follow with a good conditioner.

49

For soft, sassy waves

apply styling lotion to dry hair and

tong in large sections.

Finish by running through a little

moulding wax with your fingers rather

than brushing.

50

Changing your hair colour is one of the fastest ways to give you a completely new look and is a **great confidence booster** too.

Linda Buttle

Linda Buttle is a freelance Photojournalist who specialises in writing health, beauty and travel features for a variety of magazines and websites.

First title in the Ruby Books Beauty Series. Published 2005:

LITTLE BOOK OF
NAIL TIPS

Get the length, get the strength! Fast fixes, long

lasting gloss and how to get the best from your

manicure. Follow these invaluable tips and you'll

soon have beautiful nails.

ISBN 0 954987 10 1